Herbs For Everyday Wellness

Totally Natural Remedies For Common Ailments

Sophia Greenwood

© 2024

Copyright © 2024

All rights reserved. No part of this book may be reproduced in any form without permission in writing from the author. Reviewers may quote brief passages in reviews.

Disclaimer

No part of this publication may be reproduced or transmitted in any form or by any means, mechanical or electronic, including photocopying or recording, or by any information storage and retrieval system, or transmitted by email without permission in writing from the publisher.

While all attempts and efforts have been made to verify the information held within this publication, neither the author nor the publisher assumes any responsibility for errors, omissions, or opposing interpretations of the content herein.

This book is for entertainment purposes only. The views expressed are those of the author alone, and should not be taken as expert instruction or commands. The reader of this book is responsible for his or her own actions when it comes to reading the book.

Adherence to all applicable laws and regulations, including international, federal, state, and local governing professional licensing, business practices, advertising, and all other aspects of doing business in the US, Canada, or any other jurisdiction is the sole responsibility of the purchaser or reader.

Neither the author nor the publisher assumes any responsibility or liability whatsoever on the behalf of the purchaser or reader of these materials. Any received slight of any individual or organization is purely unintentional.

Introduction

Let's be real—life is full of little bumps in the road. Whether it's a nagging headache, a stressful day, an upset stomach, or a cold that just won't quit, we all deal with everyday ailments that slow us down. It's so easy to grab a bottle of pills or pop into the drugstore for a quick fix, but have you ever wondered if there's a more natural way to handle these issues? Spoiler alert: there totally is. Enter herbs—nature's original medicine cabinet.

Herbs have been used for thousands of years across cultures to heal and nurture our bodies. Long before modern pharmaceuticals, people relied on the power of plants to stay healthy, treat illness, and manage the wear and tear of daily life. And while there's absolutely a place for modern medicine, there's something pretty magical about turning to herbs to support your wellness in a way that feels gentle, effective, and totally natural.

I get it—herbal medicine can seem overwhelming at first. Maybe you've dabbled with a cup of chamomile tea here or some peppermint for a stomachache there, but the idea of making your own herbal remedies? That can feel like a lot. The good news? It doesn't have to be. The goal of this book is to show you how easy it can be to incorporate herbs into your everyday life, no matter your level of experience.

This isn't about ditching everything in your medicine cabinet overnight. It's about learning how to lean on nature for those common, everyday issues that pop up—whether it's calming anxiety, boosting your immune system, or simply finding relief from a headache. By the end of this book, you'll be whipping up your own teas, tinctures, and salves like a pro, with a deeper understanding of how these natural remedies can support your health.

In the pages ahead, we'll explore how to use herbs for common issues like colds, digestive problems, stress, and more. Don't worry, it's not complicated—I'll walk you through everything step by step. Whether you're growing your own herbs, purchasing dried herbs from a trusted source, or simply curious about how to get started, you'll find practical, easy-to-follow tips here that will help you feel confident in using herbs.

Let's take the mystery out of herbal medicine and get back to basics. Herbs are gentle yet powerful tools that can support your health and wellness in a way that feels natural, sustainable, and—dare I say it—pretty fun.

Ready to get started? Grab a cup of tea, settle in, and let's explore the wonderful world of herbs for everyday wellness together. You've got this!

The Power of Herbal Medicine in Your Everyday Life

Let's face it—life is hectic. From juggling work, family, and social commitments to trying to carve out a little time for yourself, it often feels like there's barely a moment to breathe. And when everyday health issues like stress, poor digestion, or colds strike, it's all too easy to reach for over-the-counter remedies without a second thought. But what if there was a more natural, balanced way to care for your health—one that aligns with the rhythms of nature and supports your body's ability to heal itself?

That's where herbal medicine comes in.

Herbs have been used for centuries, long before pharmacies existed. Our ancestors relied on the power of plants to treat everything from coughs and colds to stress and digestive issues. And here's the good news: you don't need to be an expert or a seasoned herbalist to benefit from these time-tested remedies. Incorporating herbs into your daily life can be as simple as brewing a cup of tea, adding a soothing oil to your bath, or growing a few herbs in a pot on your windowsill.

So, why turn to herbs? For one, herbal remedies are gentle but powerful. They support your body's natural healing processes, rather than masking symptoms like many modern medications. Herbs can help strengthen your immune system, reduce inflammation, calm your nervous system, and even improve digestion. And because they're natural, they often come with fewer side effects than pharmaceuticals.

But it's not just about healing when you're sick—herbs can play an essential role in your overall wellness, helping you maintain balance and vitality even when life gets chaotic. Imagine reaching for a cup of calming chamomile tea after a stressful day, or using a soothing lavender salve on irritated skin. Herbal medicine empowers you to take control of your well-being in a way that's sustainable, natural, and deeply nourishing.

In this book, we're going to explore how you can start using herbs in simple, practical ways to treat everyday ailments and support your health. You'll learn how to make teas, tinctures, salves, and more, using herbs that are easy to find and incorporate into your routine. Whether you're dealing with stress, poor sleep, digestive issues, or just want to give your immune system a little boost, there's an herb that can help.

Herbal medicine isn't just for those deep in the world of holistic health—it's for everyone. You don't need a green thumb or a degree in herbalism to start seeing the benefits of these natural remedies. With just a handful of herbs and a bit of knowledge, you can begin to make small, meaningful changes in how you approach your health.

Assembling Your Personal Herbal Toolkit

Before we dive into the world of specific remedies and treatments, you're going to need a solid herbal toolkit. Think of this as your personal collection of healing plants, oils, and supplies that will help you craft remedies whenever the need arises. Building your herbal toolkit isn't complicated or expensive, but it does require some thought about which herbs, tools, and ingredients are most useful for your needs. Once you've got the basics in place, you'll be ready to make herbal teas, tinctures, salves, and more.

I remember when I first started gathering my own herbal supplies—it was so exciting. I didn't have much space or money, but even with just a few jars of dried herbs, a tea infuser, and a bottle of olive oil, I felt empowered. I knew that I had the tools to make my own remedies, right in my kitchen. And that's exactly what this chapter is all about—helping you get the basics together so you can start making simple, effective herbal remedies at home.

Let's get started with the essentials.

Step 1: Choosing Your Starter Herbs

The first step in assembling your toolkit is picking which herbs to start with. There are thousands of herbs out there, but you don't need a huge variety to begin. In fact, just a few versatile herbs can cover a wide range of everyday health issues. Here's a list of some of the most useful and easy-to-find herbs to consider:

Chamomile: A gentle herb with calming properties, chamomile is perfect for stress relief, improving sleep, and soothing digestive issues. It's a great all-rounder and a must-have for beginners.

Peppermint: Peppermint is amazing for digestive issues like bloating, gas, and indigestion. It's also refreshing and can be used for headaches or sinus relief when you need a little wake-up.

Lavender: This aromatic herb is perfect for calming anxiety, promoting restful sleep, and soothing skin irritations. It can be used in teas, baths, and even as an oil for relaxation.

Ginger: Known for its warming and anti-inflammatory properties, ginger is great for digestion, nausea, and colds. Whether used in tea or tinctures, it adds a kick that's both healing and energizing.

Calendula: An excellent herb for skin healing, calendula is used in salves and oils to soothe minor cuts, burns, and rashes. It's also great for calming inflamed skin.

Echinacea: Known for its immune-boosting properties, echinacea is the go-to herb for cold and flu season. It's perfect for tinctures and teas that help fend off illness.

Thyme: Besides being a great culinary herb, thyme is wonderful for respiratory issues and colds. It's antibacterial and antiviral, making it ideal for fighting infections.

You can find these herbs at health food stores, online suppliers, or even grow some of them yourself if you have the space. Start with a handful of these basics, and you'll be ready to tackle a wide range of common ailments.

Step 2: Gathering Your Supplies

Now that you've chosen your starter herbs, you'll need a few tools to prepare and store your remedies. Don't worry—you won't need a ton of specialized equipment. Most of what you need can be found in your kitchen or easily purchased at a low cost. Here are the essentials:

Glass Jars: You'll need a few airtight glass jars to store your dried herbs. Mason jars work great for this. They come in various sizes and are perfect for keeping herbs fresh for long-term storage.

Tea Infuser or Strainer: If you plan on making herbal teas (which you will!), you'll need a tea infuser or a fine-mesh strainer. A tea infuser allows you to steep herbs directly in your cup, while a strainer is handy for separating herbs from liquid after making infusions or decoctions.

Measuring Spoons: You'll need measuring spoons to measure out your herbs for teas, tinctures, or salves. It's helpful to have precise measurements, especially when you start blending herbs or making more concentrated remedies like tinctures.

Mortar and Pestle (Optional): This isn't a must-have, but it's useful for grinding up herbs, seeds, or roots before making teas or oils. I love the hands-on feel of using a mortar and pestle—there's something so grounding about preparing your herbs this way.

Glass Bottles and Droppers: If you're making tinctures or herbal oils, you'll need small glass bottles to store them. Amber or dark glass bottles are best, as they protect the herbs from sunlight, helping them last longer.

Cheesecloth or Fine Mesh Strainer: If you're making infused oils or tinctures, you'll need something to strain out the herbs once the infusion process is complete. Cheesecloth or a fine-mesh strainer works well for this.

Labels: It's easy to lose track of what you've made and when, so label everything! Use small labels or masking tape to write the name of the herb, the date you prepared it, and any special instructions for use (like dosage for tinctures).

With just these simple tools, you'll be well on your way to crafting your own herbal remedies at home.

Step 3: Making Your First Herbal Remedies

Now that you've got your herbs and tools, it's time to start making some basic remedies. Let's keep it simple to begin with—teas, tinctures, and salves are great first projects for any herbalist. Here's a quick guide to get you started:

Herbal Teas (Infusions): This is one of the easiest ways to use herbs. Simply measure out 1-2 teaspoons of dried herbs (or 2 tablespoons of fresh herbs) per cup of boiling water. Let the herbs steep for 5-10 minutes for leafy herbs or flowers, or up to 20 minutes for roots and barks. Strain, and enjoy. You can add honey, lemon, or other flavorings if you like.

Herbal Tinctures: Tinctures are more concentrated remedies made by steeping herbs in alcohol or glycerin. To make a tincture, fill a glass jar halfway with dried herbs, and cover them completely with alcohol (vodka or brandy works well). Let the herbs steep in the alcohol for 4-6 weeks, shaking the jar daily. Once ready, strain the herbs and store the liquid in a glass dropper bottle. Tinctures can be taken by the dropper full, diluted in water or tea.

Herbal Salves: To make a salve, you'll need an herbal-infused oil (which you can make by steeping herbs in a carrier oil like olive oil for 4-6 weeks) and some beeswax. Melt the beeswax (about 1 tablespoon for every 1/4 cup of oil) in a double boiler, then stir in your herbal oil. Pour the mixture into small jars, let it cool, and you've got a soothing salve for cuts, dry skin, or sore muscles.

Step 4: Organizing Your Toolkit

Now that you've gathered your herbs, supplies, and maybe even made a few remedies, it's time to organize your toolkit. A small shelf or cupboard in your kitchen can easily be transformed into your personal apothecary. Store your dried herbs in glass jars, label them clearly, and keep your oils, tinctures, and salves within easy reach.

You don't need a massive setup—a few well-chosen herbs and supplies can go a long way in taking care of your everyday wellness. And as you get more comfortable with herbal medicine, your toolkit will grow naturally. You'll find yourself adding new herbs, experimenting with different remedies, and creating your own blends to suit your needs.

Once you have your herbal toolkit in place, you'll be ready to tackle common health issues with confidence, knowing you have everything you need to craft natural, effective remedies.

Herbal Remedies For Your Digestive Health

We've all been there—those uncomfortable moments when your stomach's in knots, you've overindulged at dinner, or things just aren't, well, moving along as they should. Digestion can be a tricky part of health to manage, especially with our busy lives, but the good news is that herbs offer gentle, natural solutions to many common digestive issues. Whether it's bloating, indigestion, nausea, or irregularity, herbs can support and soothe your digestive system in ways that are easy to incorporate into your daily routine.

In this chapter, we'll dive into some of the most effective herbal remedies for improving digestion, relieving discomfort, and supporting overall gut health. These remedies can be as simple as brewing a cup of tea or making a soothing tincture. Let's explore the herbs that can help get your digestion back on track.

Understanding Digestive Health

Before we get into the herbs, let's talk briefly about why digestive health matters. Your digestive system is responsible for breaking down food, absorbing nutrients, and eliminating waste. When it's functioning well, you feel energized and balanced. But when it's not, you can experience bloating, indigestion, gas, constipation, diarrhea, or even fatigue.

A healthy gut isn't just about avoiding discomfort—it's essential for overall well-being. It plays a key role in your immune system, mood, and energy levels. Herbal remedies can support this process by soothing the digestive tract, reducing inflammation, and stimulating healthy digestion.

Common Digestive Issues and Their Herbal Solutions

Indigestion and Heartburn

Indigestion, or dyspepsia, is that uncomfortable burning or bloating feeling in your stomach after eating, often accompanied by heartburn. Certain herbs can help calm the digestive tract, neutralize stomach acid, and ease discomfort.

Peppermint: One of the best-known herbs for soothing indigestion and heartburn, peppermint helps relax the muscles of the digestive tract and can relieve gas, bloating, and nausea. A cup of peppermint tea after a meal works wonders for easing discomfort.

Ginger: Ginger is a powerful digestive aid that stimulates digestion, reduces inflammation, and soothes the stomach. Whether you're dealing with nausea, gas, or indigestion, ginger tea or fresh ginger in food is a great go-to.

Fennel: Known for its carminative properties (meaning it helps reduce gas), fennel is excellent for calming bloating and heartburn. You can chew on fennel seeds after a meal or make a fennel tea to ease discomfort.

Simple Peppermint Tea Recipe for Indigestion:

- 1 teaspoon dried peppermint leaves (or 2 teaspoons fresh)
- 1 cup boiling water
- Steep for 5-10 minutes, then sip slowly after meals to calm your digestive system.

Gas and Bloating

Gas and bloating are common digestive complaints, often caused by eating too fast, poor food combinations, or certain foods that don't sit well in your stomach. The good news? Several herbs can help dispel gas and ease bloating.

Caraway: Caraway seeds are great for relieving bloating and gas by stimulating the digestive tract and reducing spasms. You can chew on a few seeds after meals or brew a tea from the seeds.

Chamomile: Known for its calming effects, chamomile also helps relax the digestive system, making it an excellent choice for relieving bloating and gas. Its gentle nature makes it a great option for children, too.

Dandelion Root: Dandelion root is a digestive bitter, which means it stimulates digestive juices and improves digestion, reducing the likelihood of bloating. Dandelion root tea is slightly bitter but highly effective.

Nausea and Motion Sickness

Nausea can hit at the most inconvenient times, whether it's from food poisoning, pregnancy, or motion sickness. Fortunately, there are herbs that can quickly calm an upset stomach.

Ginger: Ginger is hands-down the best herb for nausea and motion sickness. It works by promoting healthy digestion and reducing inflammation in the stomach. Ginger tea or even small slices of raw ginger can help settle your stomach quickly.

Peppermint: Peppermint's cooling and calming effect is perfect for soothing nausea, whether it's from digestive upset or motion sickness. A cup of peppermint tea can be sipped slowly to ease discomfort, or you can carry peppermint essential oil for quick relief—just inhale or dab a bit on your wrist.

Lemon Balm: A gentle herb, lemon balm is known for calming both the mind and digestive system. It's particularly good for easing nausea caused by stress or anxiety. Sip on lemon balm tea or combine it with ginger for extra potency.

Constipation and Irregularity

When things aren't moving as smoothly as they should, constipation can leave you feeling sluggish and uncomfortable. Certain herbs can gently stimulate digestion and get things back on track.

Senna: Known for its strong laxative effect, senna is a powerful herb for relieving constipation. However, it should be used sparingly, as it can cause cramping if taken in excess. Senna tea is a quick remedy for occasional constipation.

Psyllium Husk: Psyllium husk is a natural source of fiber that helps bulk up the stool and ease its passage through the digestive tract. It's gentle and can be used regularly to promote healthy bowel movements. Mix psyllium husk powder with water or juice and drink quickly.

Flaxseed: Another gentle source of fiber, flaxseed helps lubricate the digestive tract and ease constipation. You can sprinkle ground flaxseed on your food, add it to smoothies, or soak it in water to drink.

Diarrhea

On the opposite end of the spectrum, diarrhea can be equally disruptive. Fortunately, herbs can help calm the digestive tract and restore balance.

Chamomile: Chamomile's anti-inflammatory and soothing properties make it a great choice for calming diarrhea and settling the stomach. Sip on chamomile tea to reduce inflammation and ease cramping.

Blackberry Leaf: Blackberry leaf is an astringent herb that helps tighten tissues and reduce excessive bowel movements. A tea made from dried blackberry leaves is a traditional remedy for diarrhea and works well to firm up stools.

Slippery Elm: Slippery elm forms a soothing gel-like substance when mixed with water, which helps coat the digestive tract and relieve irritation. It's great for calming inflammation and promoting healing during bouts of diarrhea.

Everyday Tips for Digestive Health

While herbs are powerful allies for digestive issues, there are a few lifestyle habits you can adopt to support your gut health on a daily basis.

Eat Slowly: Taking your time to chew food thoroughly aids digestion and helps prevent overeating, which can lead to bloating and discomfort.

Stay Hydrated: Drinking plenty of water throughout the day supports healthy digestion and helps prevent constipation.

Incorporate Bitters: Herbal bitters (like dandelion root, gentian, or burdock) stimulate digestion and help prevent sluggish digestion and bloating. Try adding a few drops of bitters to water before meals.

Limit Processed Foods: Foods that are high in fat, sugar, or additives can slow digestion and lead to issues like constipation, gas, or heartburn. Focus on whole, nutrient-dense foods to keep your digestive system happy.

Herbs For Stress, Anxiety, and Emotional Balance

Let's be real, stress and anxiety are just part of modern life. Whether it's juggling work, family, or dealing with life's unexpected curveballs, we all get overwhelmed sometimes. But while we can't always control the chaos around us, we *can* support our minds and bodies in dealing with it. For me, that's where herbs have become an absolute lifesaver.

Herbs have been used for centuries to help calm the nervous system, ease anxiety, and restore emotional balance. The amazing thing about herbs is that they're gentle, but powerful. They work in harmony with your body, helping you feel more grounded without totally knocking you out. Whether you're looking for something to help with everyday stress, persistent anxiety, or even to lift your mood, there's an herb that can support you.

When I first started using herbs for stress, I was dealing with a lot—racing thoughts, sleepless nights, and that constant feeling of being on edge. Finding herbs that worked for me was a game changer, and now I want to share that knowledge with you. Let's dive into some of the best herbs for managing stress, anxiety, and emotional well-being, and how you can easily incorporate them into your daily routine.

Understanding Stress and Anxiety

First, let's talk about what's going on in your body when you're stressed or anxious. When you're stressed, your body releases hormones like cortisol and adrenaline, which kickstart the "fight or flight" response. This can be helpful in short bursts, but when stress becomes chronic, it can leave you feeling frazzled and exhausted. I've been there—the constant tension, the sleepless nights, the feeling of always being on edge.

Anxiety, on the other hand, often sticks around even when there's no immediate reason to be stressed. It can feel like a loop of worry and fear that's hard to break free from. Over time, this can wear down your emotional resilience and make it harder to handle life's challenges. But here's the good news: herbs can help you break that cycle, calming your mind and body in a natural, gentle way.

The Best Herbs for Stress and Anxiety

Lemon Balm
Lemon balm is one of my absolute favorite herbs for stress and anxiety. It's super gentle but incredibly effective at lifting your mood and calming your mind. I love to sip on lemon balm tea in the afternoon when I need to take the edge off a stressful day. It's uplifting without making you feel drowsy, and it's perfect if you're feeling mentally overwhelmed or restless.

To make lemon balm tea, just steep about 1 teaspoon of dried lemon balm (or 2 teaspoons of fresh leaves) in boiling water for 5-10 minutes. It's great on its own or blended with other calming herbs like chamomile.

Chamomile
Chamomile is probably the first herb I ever tried for stress relief, and it's still one of my go-tos. There's something so comforting about a warm cup of chamomile tea at the end of a long day. Chamomile helps calm your nervous system and is perfect if anxiety is keeping you up at night. It's also great for easing muscle tension, which I tend to carry in my shoulders when I'm stressed.

I love to keep a batch of chamomile tea ready for those moments when I need to unwind. Simply steep 1-2 teaspoons of dried chamomile flowers in hot water for 5-10 minutes. Add a little honey for extra soothing.

Ashwagandha
Ashwagandha is a powerhouse adaptogen, which means it helps your body handle stress better. When I was going through a particularly stressful period in my life, ashwagandha really helped me keep things in balance. It doesn't knock you out like some calming herbs—it just gives your body the resilience it needs to deal with whatever's coming your way. Over time, it really helps build emotional and physical stamina.

You can take ashwagandha in powdered form (great for adding to smoothies) or as a tincture. I like to take it consistently over a few weeks to really feel its effects build up.

Lavender
Who doesn't love lavender? It's known for its relaxing scent, but it's also a fantastic herb for calming anxiety and improving mood. Lavender helps relax both the mind and body, and it's especially helpful if you're feeling

overwhelmed or having trouble sleeping. I love using lavender oil in a diffuser or making a simple lavender tea in the evening to help me unwind.

For a calming cup of lavender tea, use 1-2 teaspoons of dried lavender flowers in hot water. You can also add lavender to a bath for a full-body relaxation experience—just toss in a handful of dried flowers, or a few drops of lavender essential oil.

Passionflower

Passionflower is one of those herbs that's perfect when your mind just won't shut off. If you're lying in bed, staring at the ceiling, with thoughts racing around in your head, passionflower is your friend. It's excellent for calming the nervous system and easing restlessness, especially when stress is keeping you from getting a good night's sleep.

I usually take passionflower as a tincture when I need quick relief. You can also make it into a tea—just steep 1 teaspoon of dried passionflower in hot water for 10-15 minutes.

How to Start Using These Herbs

When it comes to using herbs for stress and anxiety, the key is consistency. You don't need to take a ton of herbs at once or rely on them only when things get overwhelming. I've found that the best results come from using them regularly, even when I'm not in full-on crisis mode.

You can start with one or two herbs that resonate with you—maybe a calming tea like chamomile in the evening, or adding a few drops of ashwagandha tincture to your morning routine. See how they make you feel, and adjust as you go. You might even find that certain herbs work better for specific situations—like lemon balm for daytime stress or passionflower when your mind is racing at night.

Herbs are such a gentle, supportive way to take care of your emotional health. Once you start using them regularly, you'll begin to notice how much calmer and more balanced you feel. Trust me, once you incorporate these herbal allies into your daily life, you'll wonder how you ever managed without them.

Immune Support and Cold & Flu Remedies

Let's face it—nobody likes getting sick. Whether it's the sniffles, a full-blown flu, or just feeling run down, we all know how frustrating it is when illness slows us down. The good news? Herbs have been used for centuries to strengthen the immune system, fight off infections, and help the body recover from colds and flu. When I feel the first tickle in my throat or sense my energy dipping, I reach for my herbal remedies to give my body the support it needs to fend off whatever's coming.

Herbs can be incredible allies for both preventing illness and speeding up recovery when you do catch something. In this chapter, I'll walk you through some of the best immune-boosting and cold-fighting herbs, how to use them, and some simple recipes you can whip up at home to keep you and your family healthy all year round.

Understanding Immune Support

Your immune system is your body's first line of defense against infections. It works hard to fight off bacteria, viruses, and other pathogens that can make you sick. When your immune system is strong, it can fend off these invaders more effectively, often preventing illness altogether or shortening the duration of a cold or flu.

But when your immune system is run down—whether due to stress, lack of sleep, poor diet, or just the everyday hustle—you're more vulnerable to getting sick. Herbs can help give your immune system a natural boost, making it easier for your body to fight off infections before they take hold.

The Best Herbs for Immune Support

Echinacea

Echinacea is one of the most well-known herbs for boosting the immune system, and for good reason. It's particularly effective at preventing and reducing the severity of colds and flu by stimulating white blood cells, which are your body's natural defense against infection. I like to take echinacea at the first sign of a cold—right when I feel that scratchy throat or sniffles coming on. It works best when taken early, before the illness has a chance to settle in.

You can use echinacea as a tincture, capsule, or tea. To make a simple echinacea tea, steep 1-2 teaspoons of dried echinacea root in boiling water for about 10 minutes. Drink this two or three times a day when you feel like you're coming down with something.

Elderberry

Elderberry is one of my absolute favorite herbs for cold and flu prevention. It's a potent antiviral that can help stop a cold or flu in its tracks. Elderberries are packed with antioxidants and vitamins that support immune function, making them perfect for strengthening your defenses during cold and flu season. Plus, elderberry syrup is super easy to make, and it tastes delicious—kids love it, too!

To make elderberry syrup, simmer 1 cup of dried elderberries in 3 cups of water for about 45 minutes. Strain the berries, let the liquid cool slightly, and then stir in 1 cup of honey. Store the syrup in the fridge, and take 1 tablespoon daily for immune support, or up to three times a day when you're feeling sick.

Astragalus

Astragalus is an adaptogen, meaning it helps your body adapt to stress and strengthens your overall immune system. It's particularly good for long-term immune support, helping to build resilience so your body is better able to handle colds, flu, and other infections. I love adding astragalus root to soups and stews during the colder months for an easy, delicious way to get its immune-boosting benefits.

You can also take astragalus as a tea or tincture. For tea, simmer 1 tablespoon of dried astragalus root in 2 cups of water for about 20 minutes. Drink this regularly, especially during cold and flu season.

Garlic

Garlic is a powerhouse when it comes to fighting off infections. It's antimicrobial, antiviral, and antifungal, making it one of the best herbs for supporting the immune system and fighting off colds and flu. The key to getting the most out of garlic is to use it raw, as cooking can reduce its potency.

If you can handle it, chewing on a raw garlic clove or crushing it and mixing it with honey is a potent remedy for cold and flu symptoms. If that's too intense, you can add raw garlic to salad dressings, dips, or sprinkle it over food.

Ginger

Ginger is warming, anti-inflammatory, and has been used for centuries to support the immune system. It's particularly helpful for fighting off respiratory infections, and it also soothes nausea, making it perfect when you're feeling queasy. Ginger tea is one of the easiest ways to enjoy its benefits, and it's a great herb to combine with others like echinacea or elderberry for an extra immune boost.

To make ginger tea, slice a 1-inch piece of fresh ginger root and simmer it in 2 cups of water for 10-15 minutes. Add honey and lemon to taste, and sip throughout the day.

Herbal Remedies for Cold & Flu Symptoms

Once a cold or flu sets in, herbs can help ease symptoms and speed up recovery. Here are some of the best herbs for treating specific symptoms, like congestion, coughs, and sore throats.

Thyme

Thyme is an excellent herb for respiratory infections. It's antibacterial, antiviral, and helps loosen mucus, making it easier to breathe. Thyme tea or steam inhalation is perfect for clearing up congestion and soothing a cough.

For a steam inhalation, add a handful of fresh thyme (or 2-3 teaspoons of dried thyme) to a bowl of boiling water. Drape a towel over your head and lean over the bowl, inhaling the steam for 5-10 minutes. This will help clear your sinuses and loosen any congestion.

Licorice Root

Licorice root is soothing for the throat and helps calm coughs, making it great for relieving sore throats and persistent coughs. It's also anti-inflammatory and antiviral, which helps the body recover faster. You can make a tea with licorice root by simmering 1 teaspoon of dried root in 2 cups of water for 15-20 minutes.

Marshmallow Root
Marshmallow root is fantastic for soothing a sore throat and calming dry, irritated coughs. It creates a soothing, protective coating over mucous membranes, making it perfect for those dry, scratchy throats that come with colds and flu.

To make marshmallow root tea, simply steep 1-2 teaspoons of dried root in cold water for a few hours or overnight. Strain, and sip throughout the day to soothe your throat and calm your cough.

Yarrow
Yarrow is a go-to herb for reducing fever. It promotes sweating, which can help lower a fever naturally, and it also has antiviral properties that make it a great addition to your cold and flu remedy kit. A yarrow tea can help break a fever while also supporting your body's fight against the infection.

To make yarrow tea, steep 1 teaspoon of dried yarrow in hot water for 10-15 minutes. Drink it while warm to encourage sweating.

Everyday Immune-Boosting Practices

In addition to using herbs, there are some simple everyday practices you can adopt to support your immune system and keep yourself healthy year-round.

Eat a Nutrient-Dense Diet: Focus on whole, unprocessed foods rich in vitamins and minerals, especially fruits and vegetables that are high in vitamin C, like citrus fruits, bell peppers, and leafy greens.

Stay Hydrated: Drinking plenty of water helps flush toxins from your body and supports overall immune function.

Get Enough Sleep: Your immune system relies on rest to function at its best, so aim for 7-9 hours of sleep each night.

Practice Good Hygiene: Washing your hands regularly, avoiding touching your face, and maintaining good hygiene can help prevent the spread of germs.

Manage Stress: Chronic stress weakens your immune system, so incorporating stress-relieving practices like meditation, yoga, or simply taking time to relax can make a big difference in your immune health.

How to Start Using Immune-Boosting Herbs

When it comes to herbs for immune support, consistency is key. Start by incorporating one or two herbs into your routine during cold and flu season, whether that's sipping on elderberry syrup in the morning, brewing a cup of echinacea tea at the first sign of illness, or adding garlic and ginger to your meals.

Herbal remedies are gentle but effective, and when used regularly, they can strengthen your immune system and help you stay healthy even when everyone around you seems to be sniffling. With these herbs in your toolkit, you'll be well-prepared to handle whatever cold and flu season throws your way.

Herbal Solutions For Headaches and Tension

We all know the feeling—a headache creeping up out of nowhere, that tight band of pressure around your temples, or the throbbing pain behind your eyes. Whether it's brought on by stress, tension, dehydration, or just one of those days, headaches can really put a damper on everything. Thankfully, there are herbs that can help ease headaches and relieve the tension that often accompanies them.

Herbal remedies for headaches focus on relaxing the muscles, improving circulation, and calming the nervous system. These natural solutions can be effective whether you're dealing with a mild tension headache or a more stubborn migraine. Instead of reaching for over-the-counter painkillers, which can sometimes come with side effects, herbs offer a gentle, natural way to ease discomfort and tension.

In this chapter, we'll explore the best herbs for headache relief and tension, how they work, and how you can use them in teas, tinctures, and even topical remedies to soothe the pain.

Understanding Headaches and Tension

Headaches can be caused by a variety of factors—stress, poor posture, eye strain, dehydration, or even certain foods. One of the most common types of headaches is the **tension headache**, which feels like a dull, aching pressure or tightness, often around the forehead, scalp, or neck. These headaches are usually caused by muscle tension or stress and can last for hours or even days if untreated.

Migraines are more severe and often accompanied by symptoms like nausea, sensitivity to light or sound, and throbbing pain on one side of the head. While herbal remedies can help reduce the intensity of migraines, it's important to identify triggers (like certain foods or stress) to manage them more effectively.

The good news is that many herbs can help reduce tension, calm the mind, and relieve headaches naturally.

The Best Herbs for Headaches and Tension

Peppermint
Peppermint is one of my go-to herbs for headaches, especially tension headaches. The menthol in peppermint helps relax muscles and improve blood flow, which can ease that tight, throbbing pain. One of the simplest ways to use peppermint for headaches is by applying diluted peppermint oil to your temples, forehead, and the back of your neck. The cooling sensation provides immediate relief and helps relax the muscles in your head and neck.

To make a quick peppermint oil rub, mix a few drops of peppermint essential oil with a carrier oil (like coconut or almond oil) and gently massage it into your temples. You can also drink peppermint tea to relieve tension headaches from the inside out—just steep 1-2 teaspoons of dried peppermint leaves in hot water for 5-10 minutes.

Feverfew
Feverfew is a well-known herb for preventing and treating migraines. It works by reducing inflammation and relaxing blood vessels in the brain, which can help prevent the onset of a migraine. Feverfew is best used as a preventative measure, especially if you experience frequent migraines. Taking it regularly can help reduce the frequency and intensity of attacks.

Feverfew can be taken as a tea or tincture. For tea, steep 1 teaspoon of dried feverfew leaves in hot water for 5-10 minutes. If the taste is too bitter (which it often is), you can mix it with honey or blend it with other calming herbs like lemon balm or chamomile.

Willow Bark
Willow bark is often referred to as "nature's aspirin" because it contains salicin, a compound that works similarly to aspirin in reducing pain and inflammation. It's a fantastic herb for relieving headaches, especially if they're caused by tension or inflammation. Willow bark can be used in place of over-the-counter pain relievers but with fewer side effects.

To make a willow bark tea, simmer 1-2 teaspoons of dried willow bark in 2 cups of water for 10-15 minutes. Strain and drink when you feel a headache coming on. You can also find willow bark in tincture or capsule form for easier dosing.

Lavender

Lavender is known for its relaxing properties, making it a great herb for calming stress-related headaches. Its soothing aroma can help reduce anxiety, ease tension, and promote relaxation—perfect if your headaches are triggered by stress or emotional tension. I like to use lavender in a few different ways: as a tea, in a bath, or in essential oil form.

To make a calming lavender tea, steep 1-2 teaspoons of dried lavender flowers in hot water for 10 minutes. You can also use lavender essential oil in a diffuser or add a few drops to a warm bath to unwind and relieve tension.

Ginger

Ginger is not just for digestive issues—it's also a powerful anti-inflammatory herb that can help relieve headaches, especially migraines. Studies have shown that ginger can be as effective as some over-the-counter medications in reducing migraine symptoms, thanks to its ability to block prostaglandins (compounds that cause inflammation and pain).

To use ginger for headache relief, try drinking fresh ginger tea or adding powdered ginger to warm water with honey. For tea, simmer a 1-inch piece of fresh ginger root in 2 cups of water for 10-15 minutes. Sip slowly at the onset of a headache or migraine.

Skullcap

Skullcap is a fantastic herb for calming the nervous system and easing muscle tension. It's particularly helpful for tension headaches that result from stress or anxiety. Skullcap works as a mild sedative, helping to relax both mind and body, which can relieve the tension that leads to headaches.

Skullcap is best taken as a tincture or tea. To make skullcap tea, steep 1 teaspoon of dried skullcap in hot water for 10 minutes. It pairs well with other calming herbs like chamomile or lemon balm for a soothing tea blend.

Herbal Recipes for Headache Relief

Peppermint and Lavender Headache Balm

This is one of my favorite remedies to have on hand when a headache strikes. The combination of peppermint and lavender provides cooling relief and helps relax muscle tension. Plus, it's easy to make and can be carried in your bag for on-the-go relief.

- 2 tablespoons coconut oil or another carrier oil
- 10 drops peppermint essential oil
- 5 drops lavender essential oil

Melt the coconut oil over low heat, then remove from the stove and stir in the essential oils. Pour into a small container and let it solidify. To use, rub a small amount onto your temples, forehead, and the back of your neck for soothing relief.

Willow Bark and Ginger Tea for Headaches
This tea combines the anti-inflammatory power of willow bark with the soothing effects of ginger. It's great for headaches caused by tension, stress, or inflammation.

- 1 teaspoon dried willow bark
- 1-inch piece of fresh ginger, sliced
- 2 cups water

Simmer the willow bark and ginger in water for 15 minutes. Strain and sip slowly when you feel a headache coming on.

Feverfew Tincture for Migraine Prevention
If you experience frequent migraines, keeping a feverfew tincture on hand can be incredibly helpful. Taking it daily may reduce the frequency and severity of migraines.

- 1/2 cup dried feverfew leaves
- 1 cup vodka or brandy (80-proof or higher)

Place the dried feverfew in a glass jar and cover with the alcohol. Seal the jar and let it sit in a cool, dark place for 4-6 weeks, shaking the jar daily. After 4-6 weeks, strain the herbs and store the tincture in a dropper bottle. Take 1-2 dropperfuls (about 30-60 drops) in water daily to help prevent migraines.

Lifestyle Tips for Preventing Headaches

In addition to using herbal remedies, there are a few lifestyle habits you can adopt to help prevent headaches from happening in the first place.

Stay Hydrated: Dehydration is a common cause of headaches, so make sure you're drinking plenty of water throughout the day.

Manage Stress: Chronic stress can lead to tension headaches and migraines. Incorporating stress-relieving practices like meditation, deep breathing, or yoga can help reduce headache frequency.

Watch Your Posture: Poor posture, especially when sitting at a desk or looking down at a phone, can lead to tension headaches. Be mindful of your posture, and take regular breaks to stretch and move your body.

Identify Triggers: Some foods, like chocolate, caffeine, and aged cheese, can trigger headaches or migraines in certain people. Keeping a headache diary can help you identify your personal triggers.

How to Start Using Herbs for Headaches

If you're new to herbal remedies for headaches, start simple. Try a cup of peppermint or lavender tea the next time a headache strikes, or experiment with using essential oils for immediate relief. You don't need a whole pharmacy of herbs to get started—just one or two well-chosen herbs can make a big difference in how you manage headaches and tension.

Over time, you'll find which herbs work best for your body, and you can build your own headache relief routine that feels natural, effective, and tailored to your needs. Trust me, once you start using these herbal allies, you'll never want to go back to over-the-counter meds for every headache!

Herbal Solutions For Better Sleep

There's nothing quite as frustrating as lying awake in bed, staring at the ceiling, desperately wanting to fall asleep. Whether it's stress, anxiety, an overactive mind, or just trouble unwinding at the end of the day, sleepless nights can take a toll on your mental and physical health. I've been there—tossing and turning, watching the hours tick by, and then feeling groggy and irritable the next morning. That's where herbs come in as some of the best, natural allies to help you get the restful sleep your body craves.

Herbal remedies for sleep focus on calming the nervous system, reducing anxiety, and promoting relaxation, all without the groggy side effects of over-the-counter sleep aids. When used regularly, these herbs can help you establish a more natural sleep cycle, allowing you to drift off peacefully and wake up refreshed.

In this chapter, we'll explore some of the best herbs for better sleep, how they work, and how you can easily incorporate them into your nighttime routine. From teas and tinctures to aromatherapy and herbal baths, these gentle remedies will help you sleep soundly, naturally.

Understanding Sleep and Why It's Important

Before diving into specific herbs, let's talk about why sleep is so critical for your health. Sleep is when your body and brain recharge—it's essential for repairing tissues, balancing hormones, and clearing toxins from your brain. Without enough restful sleep, everything starts to feel harder. You might notice difficulty concentrating, mood swings, weakened immunity, and even physical aches and pains. In short, sleep is non-negotiable for overall well-being.

But when stress, anxiety, or even lifestyle habits interfere with sleep, it can be tough to get the rest you need. Herbs can help by easing your mind and body into a more relaxed state, allowing you to naturally fall asleep and stay asleep.

The Best Herbs for Better Sleep

Chamomile

Chamomile is a classic when it comes to promoting relaxation and sleep. It's one of the gentlest herbs, making it a great option for anyone, including children. Chamomile works by calming the nervous system, helping to reduce anxiety and muscle tension. It's especially helpful if you tend to lie in bed with racing thoughts or wake up frequently during the night.

To use chamomile for sleep, brew a cup of tea about 30 minutes before bed. Steep 1-2 teaspoons of dried chamomile flowers in hot water for 5-10 minutes. The gentle floral taste makes it easy to drink, and you can add a little honey if you like.

Valerian Root

Valerian root is one of the strongest herbal sedatives, making it perfect for those nights when you just can't seem to fall asleep. It's particularly helpful if your sleeplessness is tied to anxiety, stress, or muscle tension, as it has a calming and mildly sedative effect. I've found valerian to be a bit of a powerhouse when nothing else seems to work.

Valerian is usually taken as a tincture or capsule because the taste of valerian tea can be quite strong (and not in a good way). If you do make a tea, steep 1 teaspoon of dried valerian root in boiling water for about 10 minutes. Drink it about 30 minutes before bed, but be aware that valerian works best when taken consistently over time.

Passionflower

Passionflower is fantastic for calming a busy mind and soothing anxiety, especially when stress is keeping you awake at night. It helps relax both your mind and body, easing you into sleep without causing grogginess the next morning. Passionflower is great for those who experience insomnia due to mental overactivity or emotional stress.

You can make a tea by steeping 1 teaspoon of dried passionflower in hot water for 10-15 minutes, or you can take it as a tincture. I love to combine passionflower with chamomile or lemon balm for an extra soothing nighttime tea blend.

Lavender

Lavender is one of the most well-known herbs for relaxation, and its gentle calming effect can help ease you into sleep. The scent of lavender alone is enough to promote relaxation—just think about how many sleep products use lavender essential oil. But it's also helpful when taken as a tea or used in an herbal bath.

Lavender tea is easy to make—steep 1-2 teaspoons of dried lavender flowers in hot water for 10 minutes. You can also add a few drops of lavender essential oil to a diffuser in your bedroom, or mix it into a carrier oil for a relaxing pre-bedtime massage.

Lemon Balm
Lemon balm is another wonderful herb for reducing stress and promoting restful sleep. It's a member of the mint family, with a light, citrusy flavor that makes it a lovely addition to nighttime teas. Lemon balm is particularly good for people who struggle with anxiety, restlessness, or irritability before bed. It has a gentle calming effect that helps ease you into sleep without making you feel drowsy the next day.

To use lemon balm, brew a tea by steeping 1-2 teaspoons of dried lemon balm leaves in hot water for 5-10 minutes. It pairs well with other calming herbs like chamomile or passionflower.

Herbal Recipes for a Good Night's Sleep

Chamomile and Lavender Sleep Tea
This simple tea blend combines the calming properties of chamomile with the soothing scent of lavender, making it a perfect drink to enjoy before bed.

- 1 teaspoon dried chamomile flowers
- 1 teaspoon dried lavender flowers
- 1 cup boiling water

Steep the herbs in boiling water for 5-10 minutes, then strain. Sip slowly while winding down for the night.

Valerian and Passionflower Tincture for Insomnia
If you're dealing with more serious insomnia, this tincture combines the potent calming effects of valerian and passionflower to help ease you into deep sleep.

- 1/4 cup dried valerian root
- 1/4 cup dried passionflower

- 1 cup vodka or brandy (80-proof or higher)

Fill a glass jar with the dried herbs, then cover completely with alcohol. Seal the jar and store in a cool, dark place for 4-6 weeks, shaking the jar daily. After 4-6 weeks, strain the herbs and store the tincture in a dropper bottle. Take 1-2 dropperfuls about 30 minutes before bed.

Lavender Sleep Spray

This lavender spray is great for spritzing your pillow or linens before bed. The scent of lavender helps calm the mind and promotes relaxation.

- 1/2 cup distilled water
- 1 tablespoon witch hazel or vodka
- 10-15 drops lavender essential oil

Combine all ingredients in a small spray bottle. Shake well before each use and lightly spray your pillow, sheets, or room before bedtime.

Herbal Sleep Bath

There's nothing more relaxing than an herbal bath before bed. This herbal bath blend uses calming herbs to relax your muscles and soothe your mind, preparing you for a good night's sleep.

- 1/2 cup dried chamomile
- 1/2 cup dried lavender
- 1/2 cup dried lemon balm

Place the herbs in a muslin bag or cheesecloth and tie it securely. Drop it into your warm bathwater and let it steep while you soak. The warm water will release the herbs' calming properties, helping you unwind and de-stress.

Everyday Tips for Better Sleep

In addition to using herbs, making a few simple lifestyle changes can help improve your sleep quality over time.

Create a Relaxing Bedtime Routine: Consistency is key when it comes to sleep. Establish a relaxing bedtime routine that includes herbal teas, reading, or meditation to signal to your body that it's time to wind down.

Limit Screen Time: The blue light emitted from phones, computers, and TVs can interfere with your body's production of melatonin, a hormone that regulates sleep. Try to turn off screens at least 30 minutes before bed.

Keep Your Bedroom Cool and Dark: A cool, dark environment is ideal for sleep. Use blackout curtains and keep the temperature slightly cooler at night to help your body relax.

Practice Deep Breathing or Meditation: Deep breathing exercises or a short meditation session before bed can help calm your mind and prepare your body for sleep.

How to Start Using Herbs for Sleep

Start by choosing one or two herbs that resonate with you. Maybe it's chamomile tea to help you unwind after a long day or a few drops of lavender oil on your pillow to set the mood for sleep. Once you find what works best for you, make it a part of your nightly routine. Herbs work best when used consistently, and over time, you'll notice that your sleep becomes deeper and more restorative.

Herbal Solutions For Skin Healing

Your skin is your body's largest organ, and it's the first line of defense against the outside world. It protects you from environmental damage, heals itself when injured, and plays a critical role in your overall health. But with everything your skin has to handle—cuts, scrapes, burns, rashes, and daily exposure to the elements—it sometimes needs a little extra support to heal and stay healthy.

Herbs are some of the best natural remedies for skin healing. From soothing inflammation and reducing scarring to fighting infections and moisturizing, there's a wide range of herbs that can help your skin heal faster and more effectively. In fact, some of the most common herbs you might already have in your kitchen can work wonders for your skin.

In this chapter, we'll dive into the best herbs for healing your skin and how to use them in simple, natural remedies like salves, oils, and washes. These remedies can be used to treat everything from minor cuts and burns to dry skin and eczema.

The Power of Herbal Skin Healing

When it comes to healing skin, herbs can work in a variety of ways. Some herbs are anti-inflammatory, helping to soothe redness and swelling, while others are antibacterial or antifungal, protecting the skin from infection. Many herbs are also rich in antioxidants and vitamins that support the skin's natural healing processes, helping to reduce scarring and improve overall skin health.

What I love most about using herbs for skin healing is how gentle they are. They don't contain the harsh chemicals found in many commercial skincare products, which means they're less likely to irritate sensitive skin. Plus, when you make your own herbal remedies, you know exactly what's going on your skin, which can give you peace of mind.

Best Herbs for Skin Healing

Calendula

Calendula is one of the best herbs for promoting skin healing. It's anti-inflammatory, antimicrobial, and soothing, making it perfect for treating minor cuts, scrapes, burns, and rashes. Calendula also stimulates collagen production, which can help reduce scarring and speed up the healing process. I love using calendula in salves and oils for its gentle, soothing properties.

To use calendula, make an infused oil by steeping dried calendula flowers in olive oil for 4-6 weeks. You can use this oil on its own or mix it into homemade salves and lotions.

Comfrey

Comfrey is another powerhouse herb for skin healing, known for its ability to promote cell regeneration. It's often used to speed up the healing of wounds, sprains, and even bone fractures (which is why it's sometimes called "knitbone"). The key compound in comfrey is allantoin, which helps regenerate skin cells and reduce inflammation.

You can make a simple comfrey poultice by mashing fresh comfrey leaves and applying them directly to the affected area. If you're using dried comfrey, steep it in hot water to soften it before applying.

Plantain

Plantain (not the banana-like fruit, but the common weed you've probably seen growing in your yard) is fantastic for skin healing. It's rich in allantoin (like comfrey) and also has antimicrobial properties, making it great for cuts, scrapes, and insect bites. Plantain can draw out toxins, which makes it particularly useful for treating skin infections, splinters, and even bee stings.

For a quick remedy, crush fresh plantain leaves and apply them directly to the skin, or make an infused oil to use in salves and lotions.

Lavender

Lavender isn't just for relaxation—it's also excellent for skin healing. Lavender's antimicrobial and anti-inflammatory properties make it useful for treating burns, cuts, and insect bites. It's also soothing for dry or irritated skin and can help reduce the appearance of scars.

You can use lavender essential oil directly on minor burns and insect bites, or infuse dried lavender flowers in oil to make a calming skin salve.

Aloe Vera

Aloe vera is famous for its soothing and moisturizing properties, making it a go-to herb for burns, sunburns, and dry or irritated skin. The gel inside aloe vera leaves is packed with vitamins, minerals, and enzymes that promote healing and reduce inflammation.

To use aloe vera, simply cut open a fresh leaf and apply the gel directly to your skin. If you don't have access to fresh aloe, you can also find pure aloe vera gel in many stores—just make sure it doesn't contain added chemicals or preservatives.

Yarrow

Yarrow is a powerful herb for stopping bleeding and speeding up wound healing. It's been used for centuries to treat cuts, scrapes, and wounds because it helps blood clot faster and prevents infection. Yarrow also has anti-inflammatory properties, making it soothing for irritated or inflamed skin.

To use yarrow for wounds, you can make a poultice with fresh or dried yarrow leaves and flowers, or make a yarrow-infused oil to apply to cuts and scrapes.

Herbal Skin Healing Recipes

Calendula and Lavender Healing Salve

This healing salve is perfect for treating cuts, scrapes, burns, and dry skin. The calendula helps speed up healing and reduces scarring, while the lavender soothes and prevents infection.

- 1/2 cup calendula-infused oil
- 1/4 cup coconut oil
- 1 tablespoon beeswax
- 10 drops lavender essential oil

Melt the calendula-infused oil, coconut oil, and beeswax together in a double boiler. Once fully melted, remove from heat and stir in the lavender essential oil. Pour the mixture into a small jar and let it cool completely before sealing. Apply the salve to cuts, burns, and dry skin as needed.

Comfrey Poultice for Wounds and Sprains

This comfrey poultice is great for treating wounds, bruises, and sprains. It helps promote healing and reduces inflammation.

- Fresh comfrey leaves (or dried comfrey, rehydrated with warm water)
- Cheesecloth or a clean cloth

Mash the fresh comfrey leaves into a paste (or soak dried leaves in warm water to soften). Spread the comfrey paste onto the affected area and wrap it with cheesecloth or a clean cloth to keep it in place. Leave it on for 15-30 minutes before removing.

Plantain Oil for Bug Bites and Rashes

This plantain-infused oil is perfect for treating bug bites, rashes, and even minor skin infections. It helps soothe irritation and draw out toxins.

- 1 cup dried plantain leaves
- 1 cup olive oil

Place the dried plantain leaves in a glass jar and cover with olive oil. Seal the jar and let it sit in a warm, sunny spot for 4-6 weeks, shaking occasionally. After the infusion period, strain the oil and store it in a clean jar. Apply the oil to bug bites, rashes, and irritated skin as needed.

Everyday Tips for Healthy Skin

Stay Hydrated: Drinking plenty of water helps keep your skin hydrated from the inside out, which is essential for healthy, glowing skin.

Eat a Nutrient-Rich Diet: Your skin benefits from vitamins and minerals found in whole foods, especially those rich in antioxidants, like leafy greens, berries, and nuts.

Keep Your Skin Moisturized: Regularly applying natural oils or herbal salves helps lock in moisture and keeps your skin soft and supple. Use herbs like calendula, plantain, and aloe vera to promote healing and soothe irritated skin.

Protect Your Skin from the Sun: Too much sun exposure can damage your skin, so make sure to protect it with natural sunscreen or wear protective clothing.

How to Start Using Herbs for Skin Healing

Start by choosing one or two herbs that resonate with you and your skin needs. If you're dealing with dry skin or minor cuts and scrapes, calendula or lavender might be perfect. If you're prone to insect bites or rashes, plantain is a great choice. Once you find the herbs that work for your skin, you can start making your own salves, oils, and poultices to keep your skin healthy, soothed, and glowing.

With these herbal remedies, you'll be ready to handle whatever your skin throws at you—naturally and gently. And trust me, once you start using these herbs, your skin will thank you!

Assembling a Herbal First Aid Kit For Your Family

Life happens. Scraped knees, burns from cooking, insect bites, rashes—you name it. Whether you're at home or on the go, having a first aid kit can make a world of difference. But what if your first response to these everyday mishaps didn't involve a chemical-filled ointment or over-the-counter pills? Instead, what if your kit was packed with gentle, natural remedies from plants that have been used for healing for centuries?

That's where the **herbal first aid kit** comes in. It's a toolkit filled with powerful yet gentle herbs that can soothe, heal, and support your family's health in a natural way. Best of all, most of these remedies can be easily made at home with just a few simple ingredients.

In this chapter, we're going to walk through the essential herbs and preparations you'll need to assemble your own herbal first aid kit. Whether you're treating a minor burn, a bug bite, or a cut, you'll be able to grab exactly what you need, knowing it's free from harmful chemicals and full of healing power.

Why an Herbal First Aid Kit?

A traditional first aid kit is important for emergencies, but herbal remedies bring something extra—they work in harmony with your body, supporting its natural healing processes. Many herbs are antibacterial, antifungal, or anti-inflammatory, which means they not only soothe and heal but also protect against infection and help wounds recover more quickly. Plus, herbal remedies are gentle, often with fewer side effects than synthetic products, making them perfect for kids and sensitive skin.

Building your herbal first aid kit will give you the confidence to handle minor injuries and ailments naturally, with safe, effective treatments that have been used for generations.

Essential Herbs for Your Herbal First Aid Kit

Calendula

Calendula is a must-have for any herbal first aid kit. It's anti-inflammatory, antimicrobial, and promotes rapid healing, making it perfect for cuts, scrapes, burns, and rashes. You can use calendula as an infused oil, salve, or even as a wash for irritated skin. It's especially great for kids, as it's super gentle and non-irritating.

Lavender
Lavender is a versatile herb that works wonders for soothing burns, insect bites, and skin irritations. Its calming scent also helps ease stress and anxiety, which can be helpful in first aid situations where emotions are running high. Lavender essential oil can be applied directly to the skin for small burns or mixed into a salve for a more soothing treatment.

Plantain
Plantain is a common "weed" that packs serious healing power. It's excellent for drawing out toxins, making it perfect for treating insect bites, stings, and minor infections. Plantain also helps stop itching and promotes faster healing. Fresh plantain leaves can be crushed and applied directly to the skin, or you can make an infused oil for long-term use in salves and creams.

Yarrow
Yarrow is known for its ability to stop bleeding and promote wound healing, which makes it essential for treating cuts and scrapes. It's also anti-inflammatory and antibacterial, so it helps prevent infections. Yarrow can be used as a poultice, tea, or tincture, and dried yarrow can be kept on hand in your first aid kit for quick use.

Comfrey
Comfrey is fantastic for promoting tissue repair, making it great for sprains, bruises, and wounds. It speeds up the healing of broken bones and deep tissue injuries thanks to its high levels of allantoin, which promotes cell regeneration. Comfrey can be used as a poultice, salve, or infused oil.

Echinacea
Echinacea is your go-to for immune support and infection prevention. It's great for treating cuts and scrapes because it boosts the immune response, helping the body fight off infections. Echinacea can be applied topically in salves or taken internally as a tincture or tea to support the immune system.

Arnica

Arnica is a great herb for treating bruises, sprains, and muscle pain. It helps reduce inflammation and promotes healing of soft tissue injuries, making it ideal for bumps and bruises. Arnica is usually used as a cream or salve and should never be applied to broken skin.

Basic Supplies for Your Herbal First Aid Kit

Now that you have your herbs, let's talk about the basic tools and supplies you'll need to put together your herbal first aid kit. Most of these items are easy to find, and many you might already have on hand:

- **Glass jars or tins**: To store salves, oils, and tinctures.
- **Amber dropper bottles**: For storing herbal tinctures.
- **Cheesecloth or fine mesh strainer**: For straining herbs from oils or tinctures.
- **Bandages and gauze**: For covering cuts and scrapes after applying herbal treatments.
- **Cotton pads or swabs**: For applying tinctures, oils, or salves to the skin.
- **Small spray bottles**: Perfect for storing herbal sprays (like lavender or calendula) that can be used on cuts, burns, or bites.

Key Herbal Preparations for Your First Aid Kit

Calendula Salve for Cuts and Scrapes

This multipurpose salve is soothing, healing, and great for all kinds of skin issues, from minor cuts and scrapes to dry skin and rashes.

- 1/2 cup calendula-infused oil
- 1 tablespoon beeswax
- 10 drops lavender essential oil (optional)

Melt the beeswax in a double boiler, then slowly stir in the calendula oil. Once fully combined, remove from heat and stir in the lavender essential oil. Pour the mixture into a small jar or tin and let it cool. Apply to cuts, scrapes, and irritated skin as needed.

Plantain and Lavender Bug Bite Remedy

This simple remedy helps soothe the itching and irritation from bug bites while also reducing inflammation.

- 1/4 cup plantain-infused oil
- 1 tablespoon beeswax
- 10 drops lavender essential oil

Melt the beeswax in a double boiler, then stir in the plantain-infused oil and lavender essential oil. Pour into a jar or tin and let cool. Apply directly to bug bites for fast relief.

Yarrow Poultice for Cuts and Bleeding

Yarrow is a go-to for stopping bleeding and speeding up the healing process for cuts and scrapes.

- Fresh or dried yarrow leaves and flowers
- Warm water

If using fresh yarrow, crush the leaves and flowers to release their juices and apply directly to the wound. If using dried yarrow, rehydrate the leaves with warm water and apply the paste to the cut. Cover with a clean cloth or bandage.

Arnica Salve for Bruises and Sprains

This arnica salve is perfect for reducing pain and swelling from bumps, bruises, and sprains.

- 1/4 cup arnica-infused oil
- 1 tablespoon beeswax

Melt the beeswax in a double boiler, then stir in the arnica oil. Once combined, remove from heat and pour into a jar or tin. Allow it to cool, then apply to bruises and sore muscles (but not to open wounds).

Herbal First Aid Kit Checklist

Here's a quick checklist to help you assemble your herbal first aid kit:

- **Calendula salve** (for cuts, scrapes, burns, and rashes)
- **Lavender essential oil** (for burns, bites, and stress relief)
- **Plantain-infused oil** (for bug bites, rashes, and minor infections)
- **Yarrow tincture or dried herb** (for cuts and bleeding)
- **Comfrey salve or poultice** (for bruises, sprains, and wound healing)

- **Echinacea tincture** (for immune support and infection prevention)
- **Arnica salve** (for bruises, sprains, and muscle pain)
- **Bandages, gauze, and cotton pads**
- **Small jars, bottles, and spray bottles**

How to Use Your Herbal First Aid Kit

Once your herbal first aid kit is assembled, you'll be ready to handle everyday injuries and ailments naturally. Whether it's applying a calendula salve to a scraped knee or using a lavender spray for a minor burn, you'll have a natural remedy on hand for nearly any situation. And best of all, you'll know exactly what's going into your family's healing process—no chemicals, just the gentle power of nature.

As you get more comfortable with your herbal remedies, you can expand your kit and personalize it based on your family's needs. Whether you're using it at home or taking it with you on hikes or trips, your herbal first aid kit will quickly become one of your most trusted tools for natural healing.

Tips on Including Herbs In Your Everyday Life

Incorporating herbs into your daily life can feel like a small but powerful way to connect with nature and support your health. You don't need to be an herbalist or even have a green thumb to make herbs a part of your routine. It's all about taking simple steps that fit into your lifestyle—whether it's brewing a soothing tea, sprinkling herbs on your food, or using herbal oils for skincare. The key is consistency and making it an enjoyable practice, not a chore.

In this chapter, we'll explore some easy and practical ways to incorporate herbs into your everyday life. Whether you're looking to boost your energy, relax at the end of the day, or support your immune system, there's a way to bring herbs into your routine that will feel natural and effortless.

Start Your Day with Herbs

Mornings are a great time to infuse your day with herbs, setting the tone for energy and focus.

Herbal Teas for Energy: Swap out your morning coffee for an energizing herbal tea. Herbs like **peppermint, ginger**, and **green tea** can give you a natural boost without the jitters. If you're not ready to give up coffee, try blending in adaptogenic herbs like **ashwagandha** or **maca** powder to help your body handle stress throughout the day.

Herbal Smoothies: If you love starting your day with a smoothie, it's a great opportunity to add some herbs. A spoonful of powdered **spirulina, maca**, or **turmeric** can enhance the nutritional value and give you a gentle energy boost. Throw in some fresh **mint** or **basil** for a refreshing flavor that complements your fruit or greens.

Herbal Tinctures: If you're short on time in the morning, taking a quick dropper of an herbal tincture can give you the same benefits as tea or smoothies. A drop or two of **ginseng** or **rhodiola** tincture in your water can help jumpstart your day and support your energy levels.

Use Herbs Throughout the Day

Incorporating herbs into your daily routine doesn't have to mean changing everything—small, mindful additions can make a big difference.

Herbal Water Infusions: One of the easiest ways to include herbs in your day is by making herbal-infused water. Add fresh herbs like **mint**, **lemon balm**, or **basil** to a pitcher of water and let it steep for a few hours. The refreshing flavor is great for staying hydrated and gives you a gentle dose of herbal goodness.

Herbal Snacks: You can easily sneak herbs into your snacks or meals. Add **rosemary** or **thyme** to roasted vegetables, sprinkle **dill** on your salads, or mix dried **oregano** into your homemade hummus. You'll get the flavor benefits while also enjoying the health-promoting properties of the herbs.

Tinctures on the Go: Keep a small bottle of your favorite tincture in your bag or at your desk for easy access throughout the day. **Lemon balm** or **holy basil** tinctures are great for stress relief, while **echinacea** or **elderberry** can be taken to boost immunity, especially during cold season. Just add a few drops to your water or take them directly under your tongue.

Herbal Rituals for Relaxation and Sleep

Evenings are the perfect time to wind down with herbs that help you relax and prepare for restful sleep. These small rituals can become a comforting part of your nighttime routine.

Calming Herbal Teas: Sipping on a cup of **chamomile**, **lavender**, or **passionflower** tea before bed can help calm your nervous system and prepare your body for sleep. If you tend to feel anxious or have trouble shutting your mind off at night, these herbs are gentle yet effective for easing you into rest. Brew a cup about 30 minutes before bed as part of your evening wind-down.

Herbal Baths: Taking an herbal bath is a great way to relax both your mind and body. You can make a simple bath infusion by adding **lavender**, **chamomile**, or **rose petals** to a muslin bag and hanging it under the faucet while you fill the tub. Add a few drops of **lavender essential oil** for extra relaxation, and soak for 20-30 minutes to unwind after a long day.

Aromatic Herbs for Relaxation: Herbs aren't just for teas and tinctures—using them in aromatherapy can have a powerful effect on your mood. Try diffusing **lavender**, **frankincense**, or **bergamot essential oil** in your bedroom to promote relaxation before sleep. You can also make a simple herbal sachet filled with **lavender** or **hops** to place under your pillow for better sleep.

Cooking with Herbs

One of the easiest and most flavorful ways to incorporate herbs into your daily life is through your meals. Fresh or dried herbs can add depth to your cooking while offering health benefits.

Herbal Broths and Soups: Adding herbs like **thyme, rosemary, sage,** and **oregano** to your broths and soups not only enhances flavor but also supports your immune system. These herbs are rich in antioxidants and have antimicrobial properties, making them perfect for cooking, especially during cold and flu season.

Herbal Oils and Vinegars: Making your own herbal-infused oils or vinegars is easy and can add a burst of flavor and healing benefits to your cooking. Infuse olive oil with herbs like **rosemary** or **garlic** and use it in salad dressings or as a dip for bread. **Herbal vinegars** can be made by steeping herbs in apple cider vinegar—**thyme** or **oregano** vinegar is great for adding to salads or sauces.

Herbs as Seasoning: Keep a variety of dried herbs on hand to sprinkle over your food. **Basil, oregano, thyme,** and **cilantro** are all versatile herbs that can be added to soups, stews, roasted vegetables, or meats for an extra boost of flavor and health.

Use Herbs for Immune Support

Herbs are also great for boosting your immune system and preventing illness, especially during colder months.

Herbal Tonics: Keep your immune system strong by incorporating immune-boosting herbs into your daily routine. **Elderberry** syrup is one of the best ways to support your immune health. Take a spoonful each morning as a preventative measure during cold and flu season. You can also make **fire cider** by steeping **garlic, ginger, horseradish,** and **apple**

cider vinegar—a shot of this tonic every day is excellent for immune support.

Tinctures for Immune Health: Herbs like **echinacea** and **astragalus** can be taken daily to keep your immune system in check. Add a dropperful of these tinctures to water or tea, especially when you're feeling run down or exposed to illness.

Skincare with Herbs

Herbs can also play a role in your skincare routine, offering soothing, healing, and nourishing properties for your skin.

Herbal Oils for Moisturizing: Herbal-infused oils like **calendula**, **lavender**, and **chamomile** are great for keeping your skin soft and moisturized. You can use them as a daily moisturizer or apply them to irritated or dry skin. These oils are gentle enough for all skin types and offer healing benefits, especially for sensitive or inflamed skin.

Herbal Face Steams: A facial steam with herbs like **rose petals**, **lavender**, or **chamomile** can help open your pores, hydrate your skin, and provide a gentle detox. Simply boil water, add a handful of herbs, and lean over the steam with a towel draped over your head for 5-10 minutes. Your skin will feel refreshed and rejuvenated.

DIY Herbal Face Masks: You can make simple face masks using herbal powders like **turmeric**, **matcha**, or **aloe vera** mixed with honey or yogurt. These masks are great for soothing inflammation, adding hydration, and giving your skin a healthy glow.

How to Start Using Herbs in Your Daily Life

The key to incorporating herbs into your everyday routine is starting small and finding what works for you. You don't need to overhaul your entire lifestyle—just begin with one or two practices that feel easy and enjoyable. Maybe it's switching out your afternoon coffee for a calming herbal tea, adding herbs to your meals, or making a nighttime routine with calming herbs like lavender or chamomile.

Over time, these small changes will add up, and you'll find that herbs naturally become part of your daily routine. Herbs are here to support you, whether you're looking to boost your energy, reduce stress, or simply enjoy the flavors and benefits they bring. Trust me, once you start using herbs, you'll wonder how you ever lived without them!

Conclusion

By now, you've seen how herbs can become powerful allies in your everyday life. Whether you're sipping on a soothing tea before bed, applying a healing salve to a cut, or using an herbal tincture to boost your immune system, these natural remedies offer gentle, effective support for your health and well-being. The beauty of herbal medicine lies in its simplicity—small, consistent steps that nurture your body in harmony with nature.

Herbal medicine isn't about quick fixes or drastic changes. It's about developing a deeper connection with the plants around you, learning to trust in the natural healing processes of your body, and taking a more mindful, intentional approach to your health. These herbs have been used for centuries across cultures for a reason—they work.

As you continue on your herbal journey, remember that it's okay to start small. Choose one or two herbs that resonate with you and gradually build from there. Whether it's through teas, tinctures, salves, or simply sprinkling fresh herbs into your meals, you're creating a personalized approach to wellness that empowers you to take care of yourself and your family, naturally.

Herbs can transform how you approach health, offering a holistic, sustainable way to stay balanced, energized, and connected to nature. I hope this book has inspired you to explore the wonderful world of herbal medicine and, most importantly, to make herbs a part of your everyday routine.

Here's to a life supported by nature, one herb at a time. Happy healing!

www.ingramcontent.com/pod-product-compliance
Lightning Source LLC
Chambersburg PA
CBHW081811250726
48653CB00010B/3898